GW01367328

BEDFORDSHIRE COUNTY COUNCIL
SOLD
BEDFORDSHIRE COUNTY COUNCIL
WITHDRAWN FOR SALE. PRICE: 50p

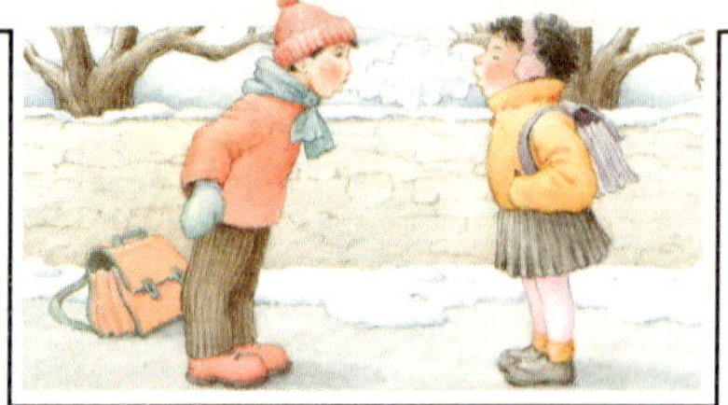

Written by Chantal Henry-Biabaud
Illustrated by Liliane Blondel

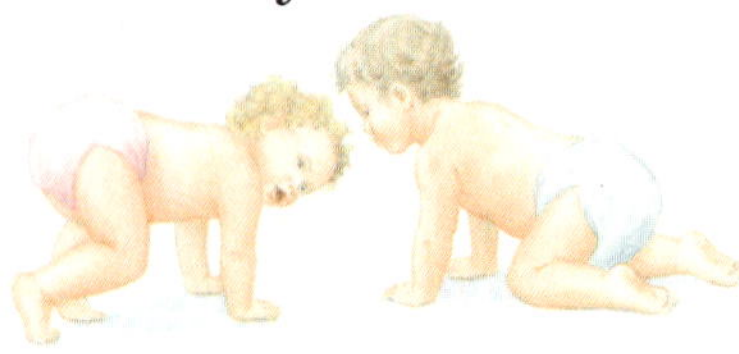

ISBN 1 85103 162 6
First published in the United Kingdom
by Moonlight Publishing Ltd,
36 Stratford Road, London W8
Translated by Sarah Gibson

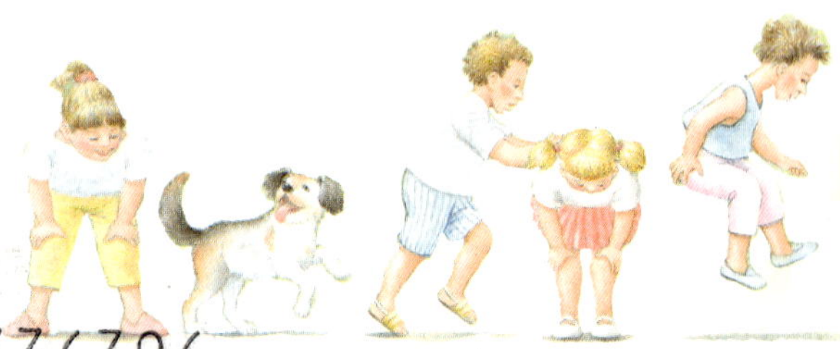

Specialist adviser:
Dr Andrew Gibson, M.B., B.Chir

Printed in Italy by Editoriale Libraria

POCKET • WORLDS

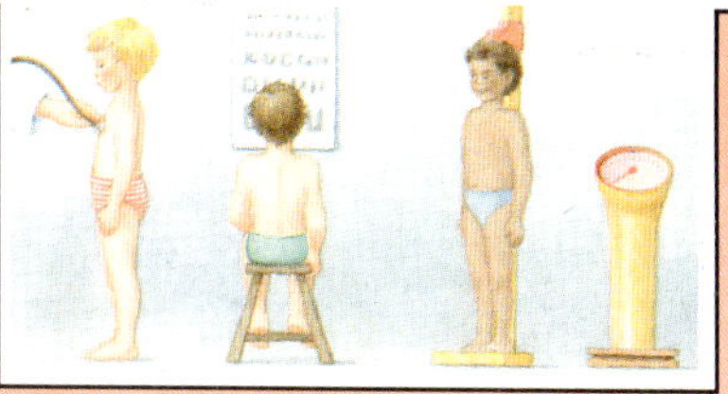

Your Body

Your body is like a fantastic machine.
Let's begin to understand
how it works!

We are all alike, yet each of us is different from everyone else.

Short or tall, fat or thin, young or old, blond, red-headed or dark, dark-skinned, coloured, black or fair-skinned, the basic model is the same.

We each have a head with hair, two eyes, two ears, a nose, a mouth; we have a body with two arms and two legs, and we are supported by a backbone to keep us upright.

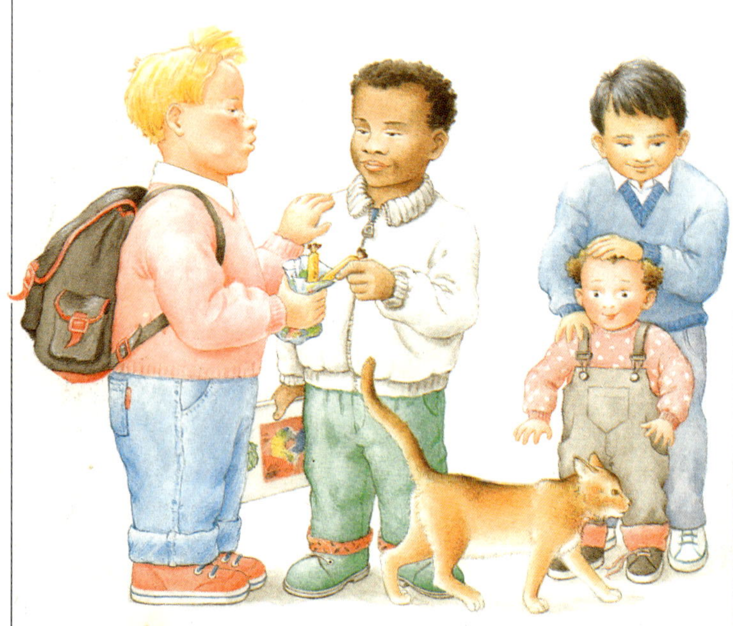

It's not just coincidence that we are all made this way.
It's because we belong to the same species, we are human beings.

It is impossible to muddle up a human being with an animal or a thing: however unusual our looks, you can always tell the difference between a child, an animal and an object!

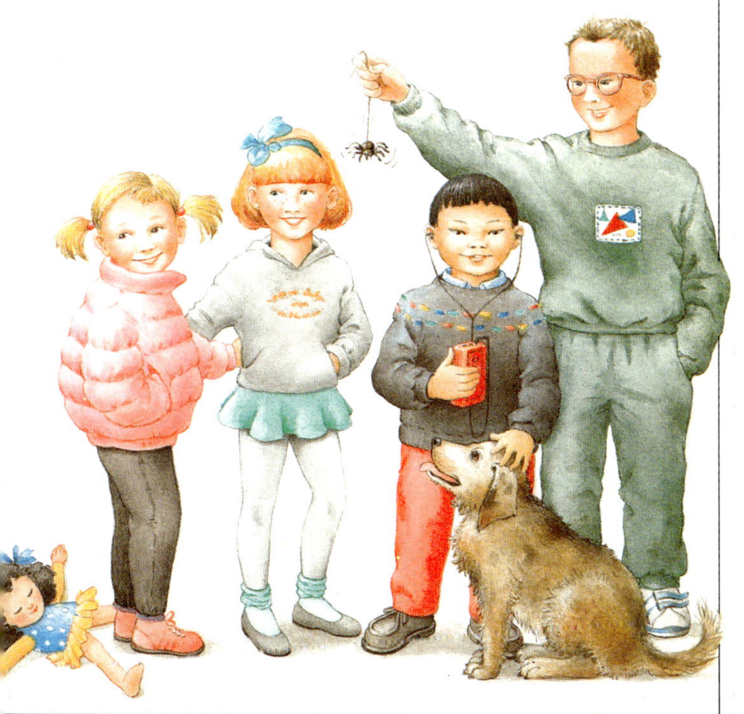

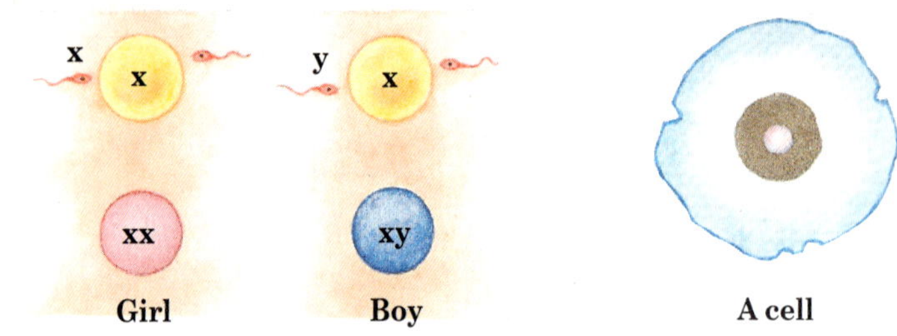

Sperm meet an ovum

Were you born a boy or a girl?

The difference is decided at the moment the baby is conceived. This is when a male and a female cell join to make a baby. The mother's cell, the egg, is an ovum. It contains a thread called a chromosome, which is always in the shape of an X. The father's cell is the sperm. Some sperms have an X chromosome, some a Y chromosome. If a sperm with an X chromosome joins the ovum, they will produce an XX cell and the baby will be a girl. If the sperm has a Y chromosome, they will produce an XY cell and the baby will be a boy. This is the first cell of your body: it will divide into two, and those two into four and so on, until many millions of minuscule cells have been formed.

The sex of an animal's babies is decided in the same way.

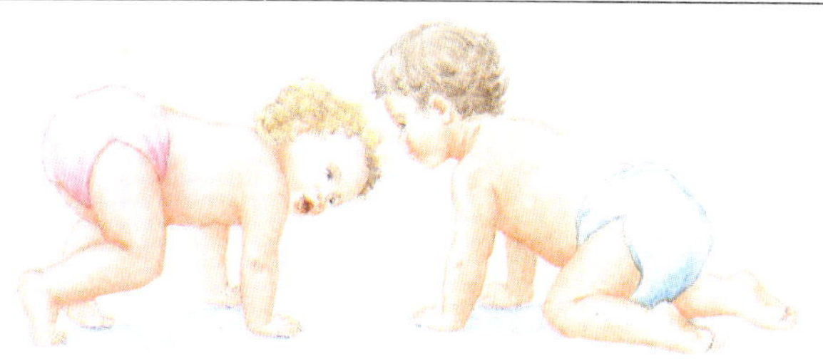

Cells are the building blocks from which everything else is made: bones, blood, muscles, skin and all the other parts of the body. Cells are programmed to organise growth and development. Grown-ups have finished growing, but their bodies change gradually over the years. Finally, like a worn-out car, the engine stops and they die. But life goes on through their children.

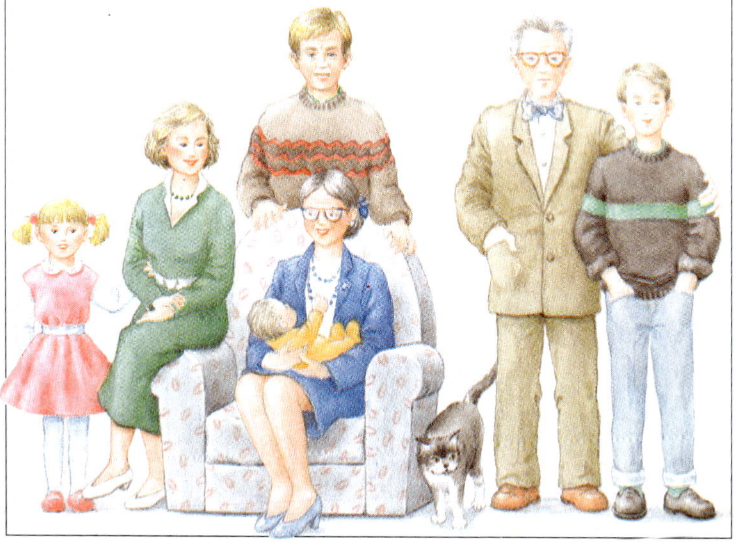

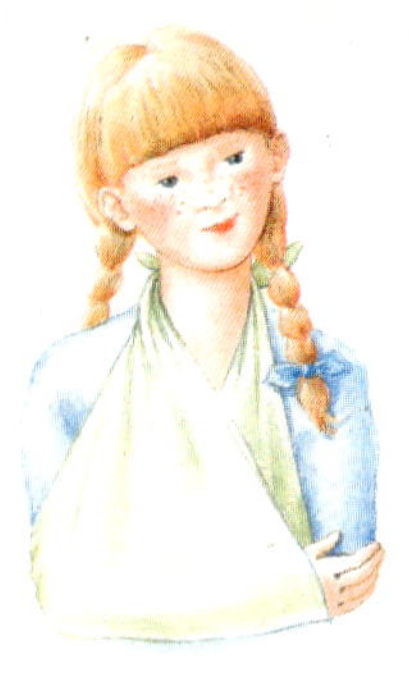

If a bone breaks, you have to plaster the limb that has fractured to keep it steady, so the bone can mend.

If you didn't have a skeleton, you wouldn't be able to stand up.

If you squeeze one of your fingers tight, you will feel something hard: it's a bone. There are more than two hundred bones in your body, of all shapes and sizes. Some have very funny names: ossicles, scaphoid, coccyx. The tiniest are inside your ear, the largest is your hip bone; others, like your teeth, don't even look like bones at all.

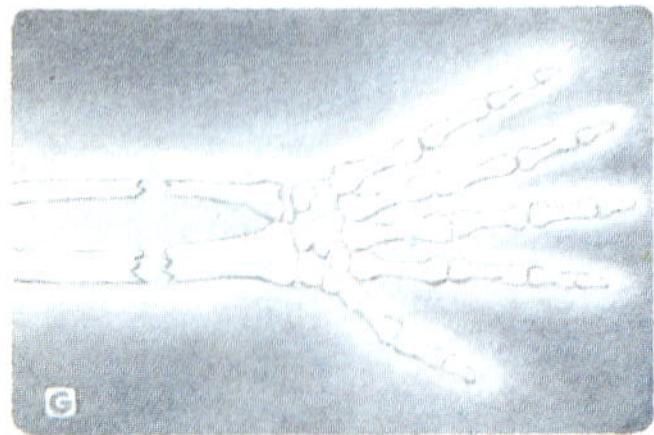

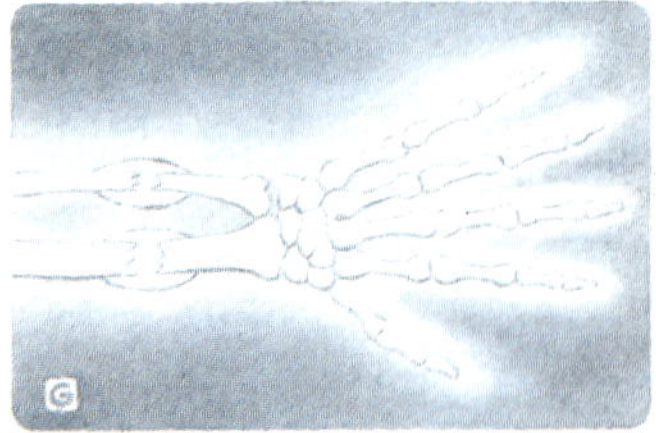

A callus forms where the bone was broken.

Your bones hold you upright, and protect your brain, your heart, your lungs and all your soft, delicate organs. Your bones make up your skeleton.

Some animals go on growing throughout their whole lives...

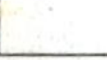

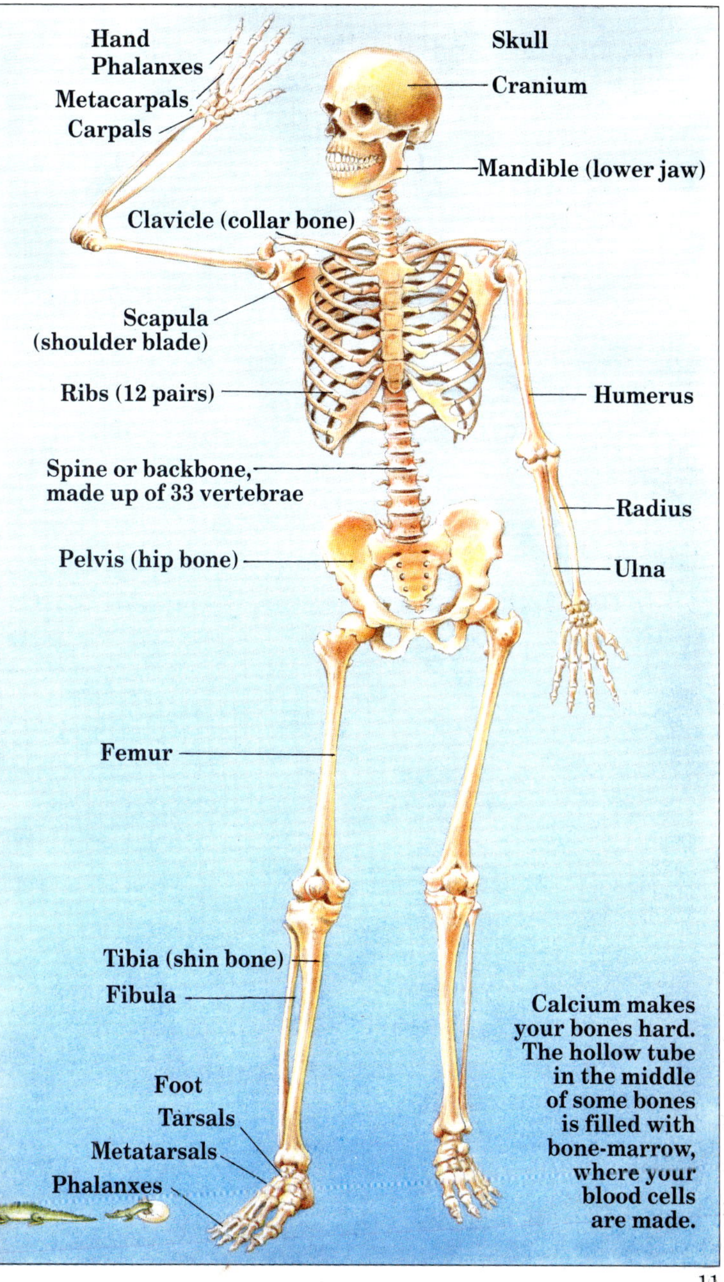

Calcium makes your bones hard. The hollow tube in the middle of some bones is filled with bone-marrow, where your blood cells are made.

Your bones can't move on their own. They need muscles to move them.

Your muscles work as they receive instructions from your brain, brought to them by nerves. You have more than six hundred muscles, big ones like those in your calves or thighs, and little ones like those which make your eyes move, or your tongue. You use the muscles of your face to smile or frown!

Your heart is a muscle too. It is controlled by nerves like other muscles, but it has an automatic mechanism which means it can beat on its own as well.

To bend your arm at the elbow, the front muscles shorten and contract, whilst the back muscles stretch and relax.

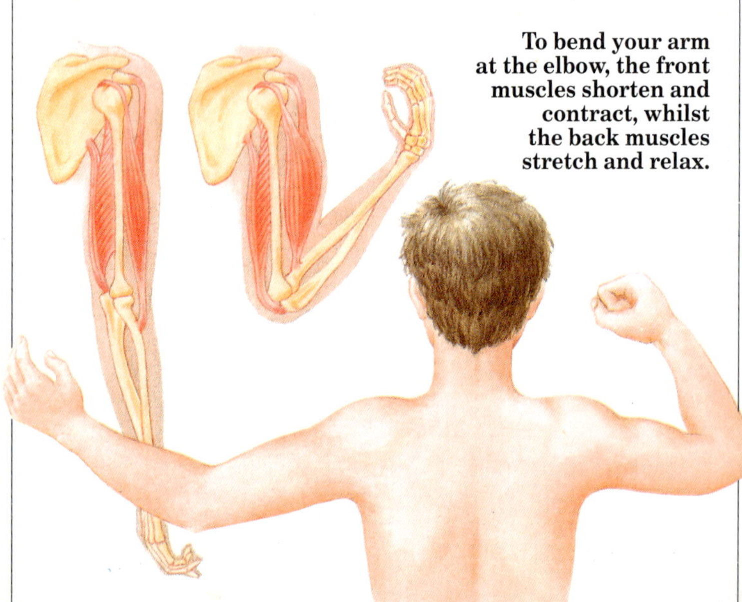

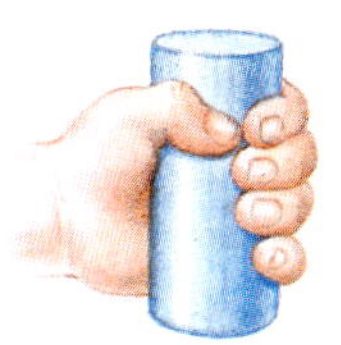

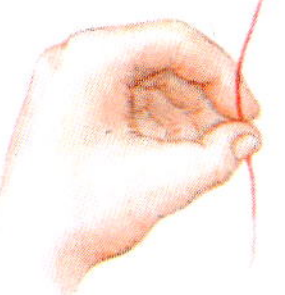

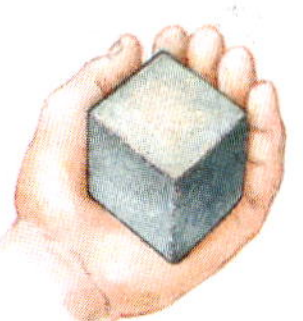

Your muscles enable you to hold things. A baby finds it difficult to pick up a thread between two fingers.

Muscles need lots of energy if they are to work properly. We eat to give us energy. Food passes into the blood and brings energy to all the cells in our bodies.

Sometimes your muscles hurt.

Do you ever feel stiff after you have overworked muscles that are not used to exercise? Or you might get cramp: this can happen when waste products build up in muscle and cause a sharp pain, warning you to rest for a while.

Tendons attach muscles to bones; ligaments hold bones and joints in position. If you pull a ligament or a tendon in your ankle or your knee, you will have a sprain.

Your skin is made up of two layers: the epidermis on top, and the dermis underneath. There are tiny holes in it called pores.

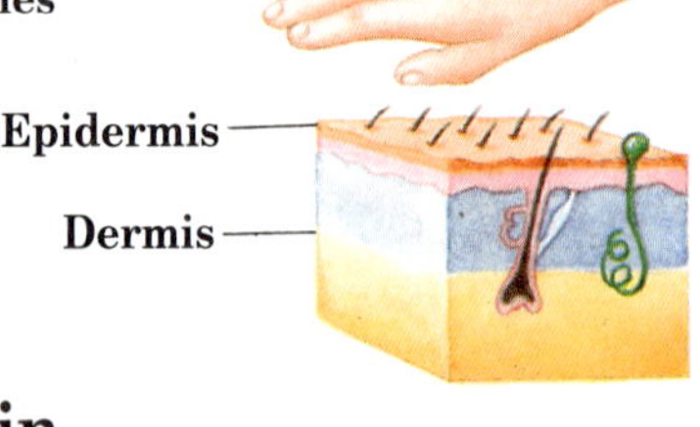

From your head down to your toes, your whole body is wrapped up in skin.

Your body contains a lot of water. If you did not have a covering of skin, the water would run out or evaporate in the air. You would look rather like a shrivelled-up prune! Your skin does not just stop water escaping, it also stops water going in. It produces a sort of grease called sebum, which makes it waterproof. If it was not waterproof, you would swell up in the bath rather like a sponge! Skin gives you good protection against germs. They can't get through if your skin is healthy.

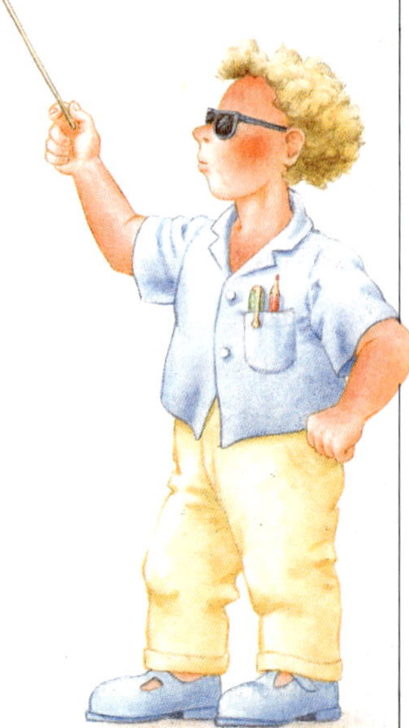

Your skin protects you against the sun, but if you are not careful your skin can get sunburned. In the summer, put on a good sun screen cream and wear a hat.

We help the skin do its work by wearing light clothes in the summer and dressing up warmly in the winter.

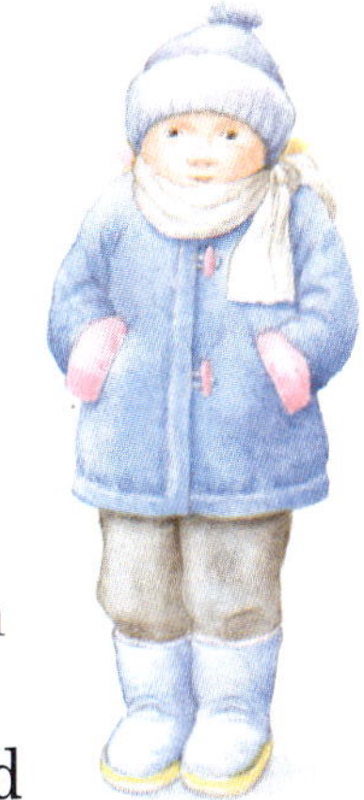

Your skin helps you adapt to hot and cold. When it's hot, little glands produce sweat, which cools you down as it evaporates. Your blood vessels open up and rise to the surface of your skin to help cool the blood. That's why you look flushed. When it's cold, your blood vessels contract to keep in heat, and the hairs on your arms and legs stand up: you've got goose pimples!

Do you like having a bath?

It's a good thing to wash, because dirt and dust stick to sebum. As you rub yourself, you take off the old layer of grease. It's replaced at once with a fresh one.

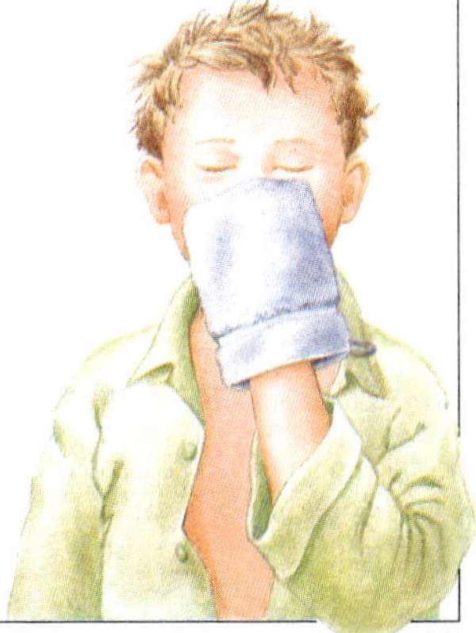

Your face is never covered up, so it needs a good wash at least twice a day.

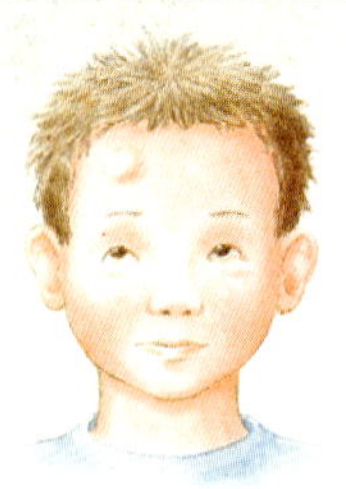

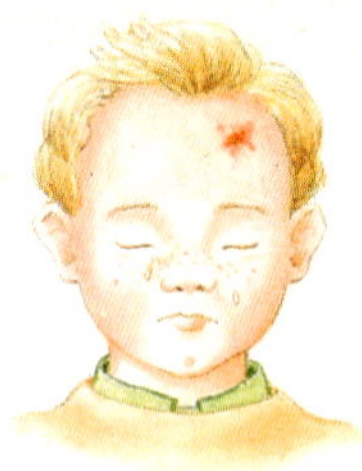

You fall over, and there you are with a bump, a graze or a bruise – and if you're really unlucky, all three at once!

Bumps and bruises

Your skin is strong, it gives you good protection. But every now and then you will have an accident. If you fall over, you may find you have a swollen lump which turns into a bruise. The blood vessels have broken and you are bleeding under the skin. Luckily, special cells rush to repair the damage, but if you are badly hurt, you might have to go to the doctor.

Be especially careful of burns and scalds. When you burn yourself, you lose your protective layer of skin and you are in danger of losing your body fluids.

Boiling water, an iron, electricity...lots of things around the house can burn you.

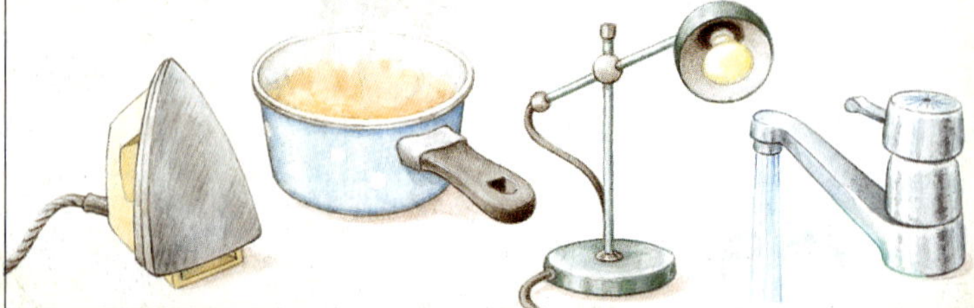

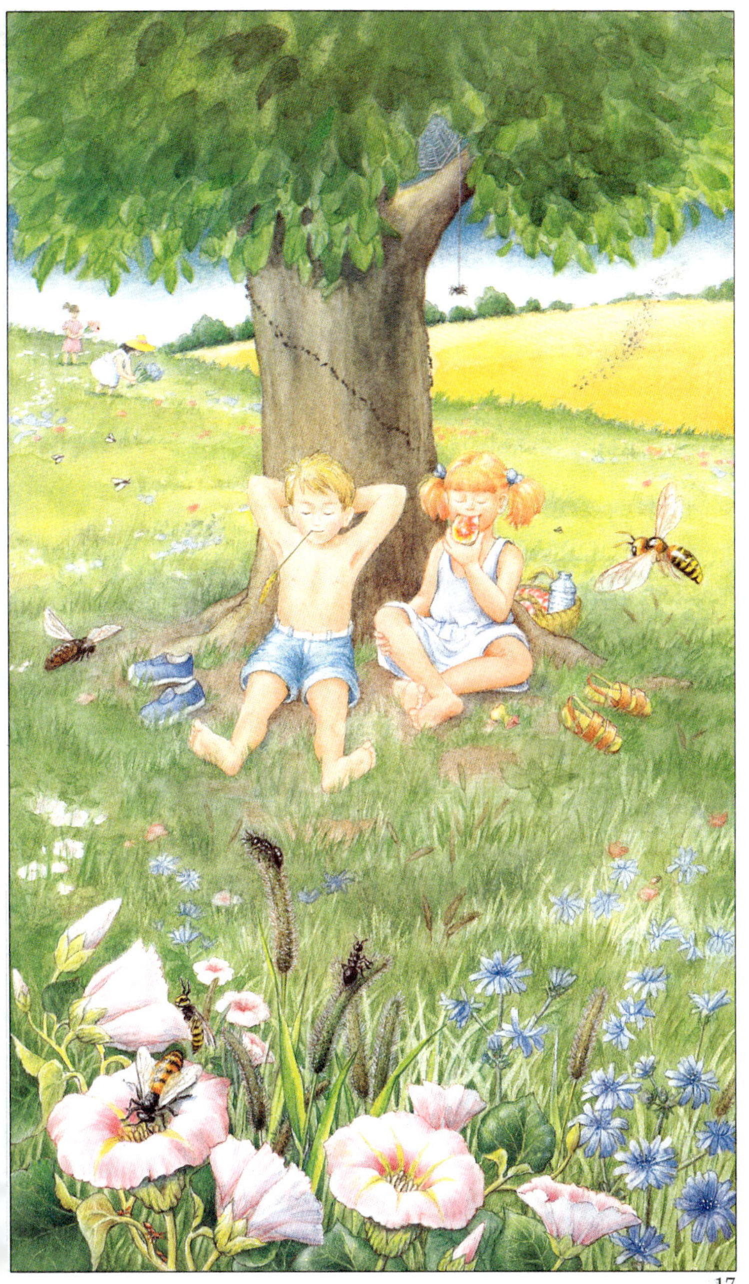

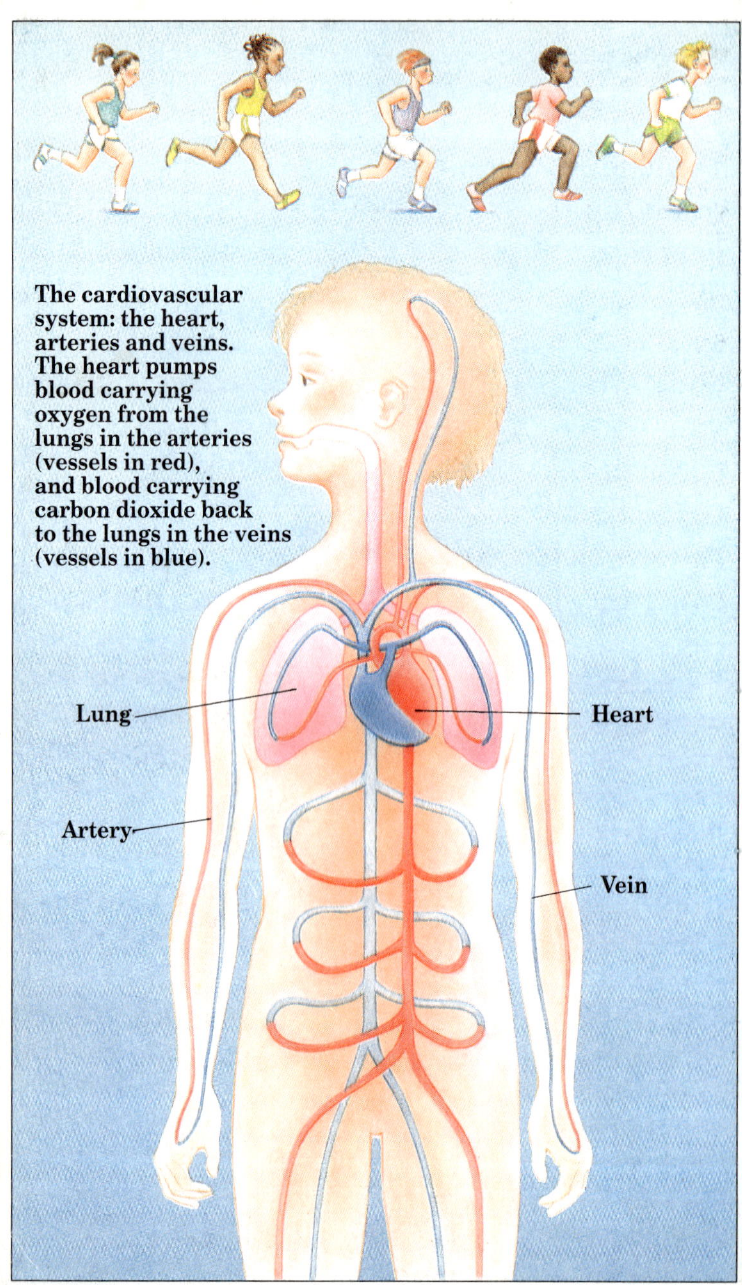
The cardiovascular system: the heart, arteries and veins. The heart pumps blood carrying oxygen from the lungs in the arteries (vessels in red), and blood carrying carbon dioxide back to the lungs in the veins (vessels in blue).
Lung
Heart
Artery
Vein

When you take your pulse, you can feel your blood throbbing as it is pushed along an artery.

Your heart is beating non-stop in your chest!

It pumps, then rests, pumps, then rests, about seventy times a minute. Its rhythm speeds up when you are active, and slows down when you are asleep. The heart is like your body's engine. It pumps blood right through your body, to your toes and fingertips. The blood goes round in blood vessels, tubes which can bend. They grow tinier and tinier the further they are from your heart.

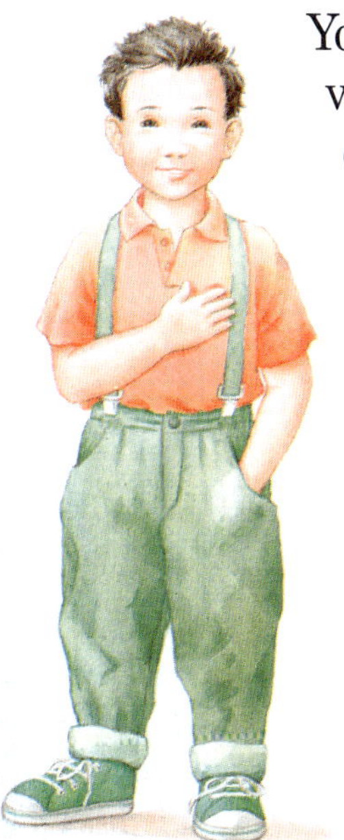

You have two types of blood vessels: arteries, which carry fresh oxygenated blood from the heart around the body, and veins which carry stale blood back to the heart. Your blood circulates in only one direction; it cannot double back.

You have 3 or 4 litres of blood in your body and it is pumped through your heart about 1,000 times a day.

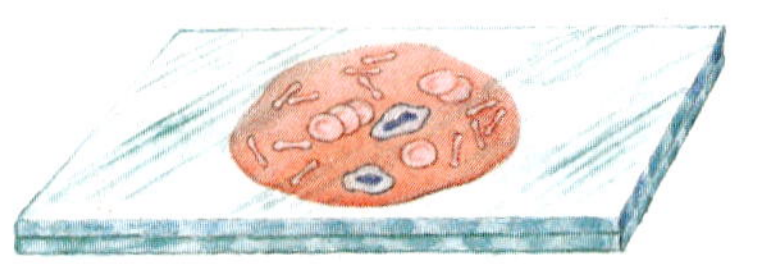

A drop of blood on a microscope slide

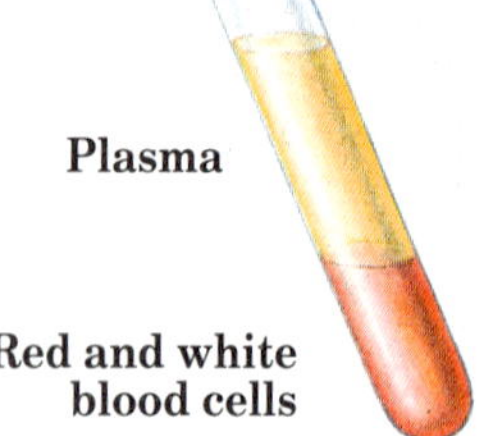

When you cut yourself, blood trickles out.

It's red and slightly sticky. It is made up of a clear liquid called plasma, in which thousands of tiny cells move about. Some are red blood cells, some are white blood cells, and some are platelets.

Each has a job to do.

Blood cells live for about three months. Red blood cells carry oxygen from the lungs to the other cells of the body. Then they take carbon dioxide back to the lungs. White blood cells fight the diseases that make us ill.

Don't scratch the scab off if you have a graze. It's there to stop germs getting in.

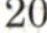

Sometimes you may get a nose bleed. This happens when a little blood vessel inside your nose is torn.

Platelets rush to block a break in a blood vessel.

As soon as you graze your knee, they are at work to repair it. The platelets bind the red cells with fibrin to form a clot that holds the blood in. As the clot dries, it turns into a scab. When the wound has healed, the scab falls off – its work is done.

Not everybody has the same type of blood. There are four different blood groups: O, A, B, AB. It is very useful to know which blood group you belong to.

Platelets collect round a wound to form a clot.

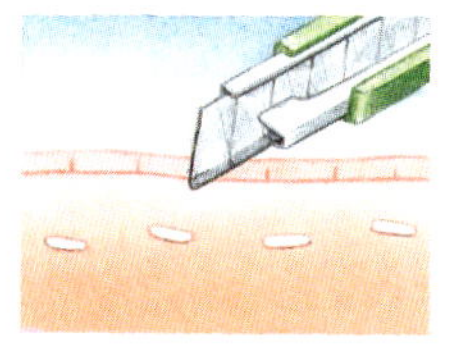

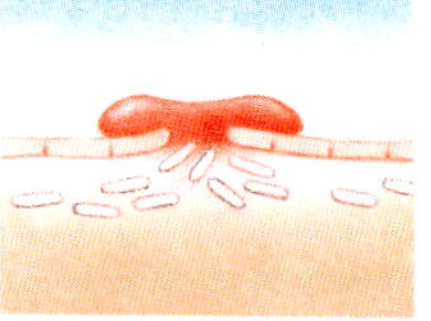

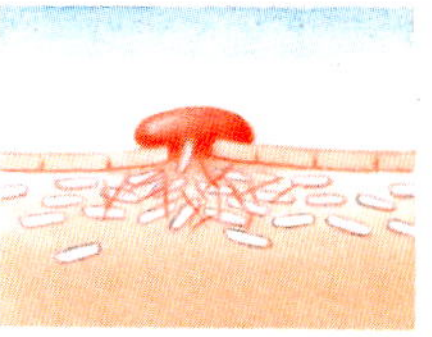

Underneath the clot, special cells repair the damage. After a few days, the cut has healed.

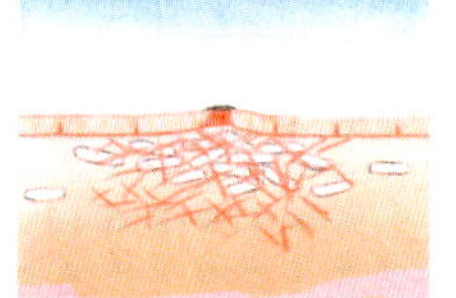

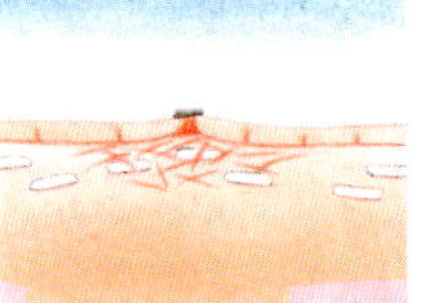

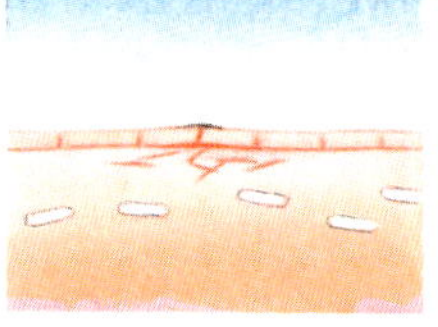

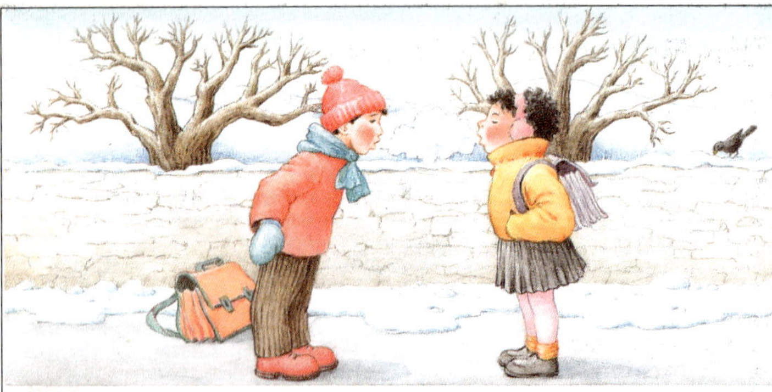

On a cold day you can see your breath, because it is warmer than the air around you and forms a cloud of water vapour.

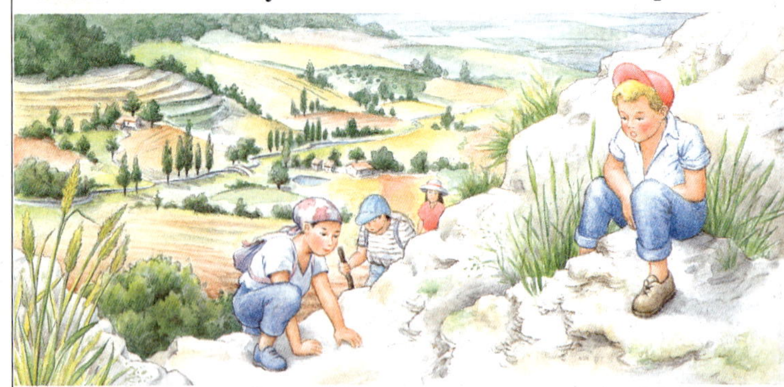

The higher you climb up a mountain, the less oxygen there is. Sometimes mountaineers suffer from mountain sickness.

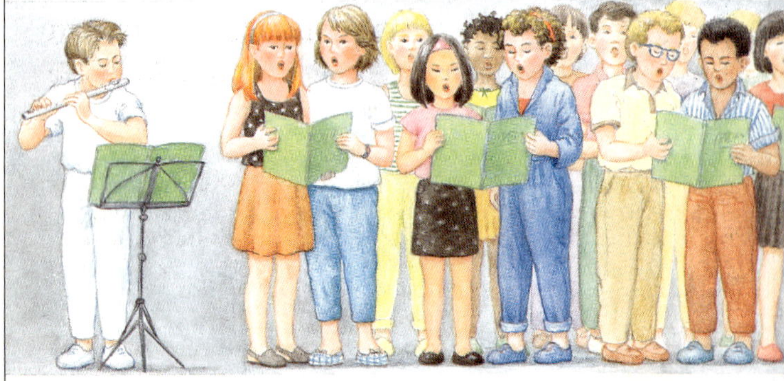

Your voice box is at the back of your throat. As you breathe out it vibrates, producing sounds: that's how you talk and sing.

The first thing a baby does when it's born is to take a great gulp of air and begin to breathe.

You haven't stopped breathing since the moment you were born.

As you breathe in, your chest expands; as you breathe out, it subsides. You breathe in two-time: in, out, in, out.

Air goes in through your nose and mouth. Inside your nose are tiny hairs to trap dirt and germs and stop them going right through the airways. Air goes down your windpipe to your lungs, where blood takes the oxygen from the air, and gets rid of its carbon dioxide and waste products. These are removed from the body as you breathe out again.

Allergies can be irritating and even painful. Some people sneeze, and their eyes go red and stream with tears when they breathe in fur or dust, or pollen from certain flowers.

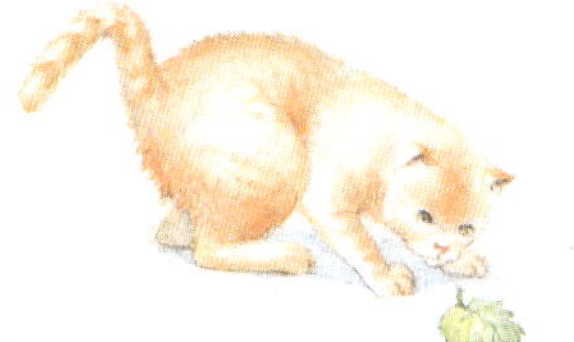

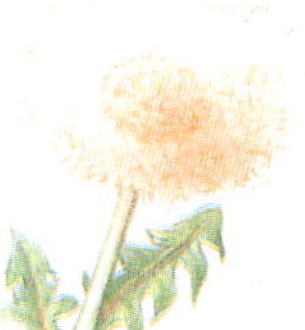

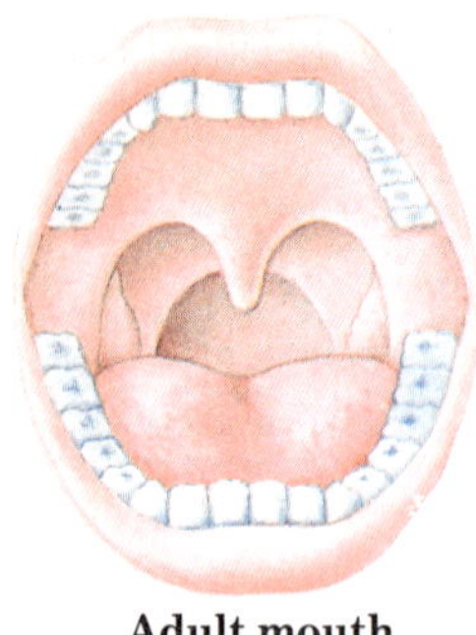

Adult mouth
with 32 teeth

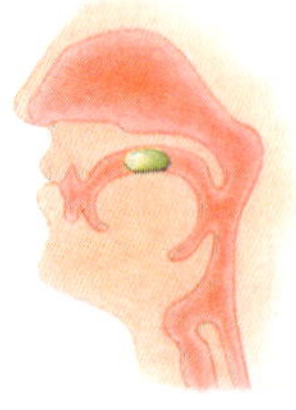

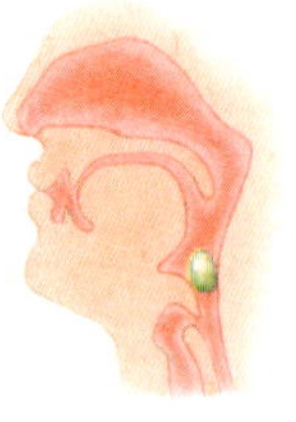

When you swallow, the epiglottis shuts off the opening to your windpipe so that food doesn't go down into your lungs.

What happens to a mouthful of food?

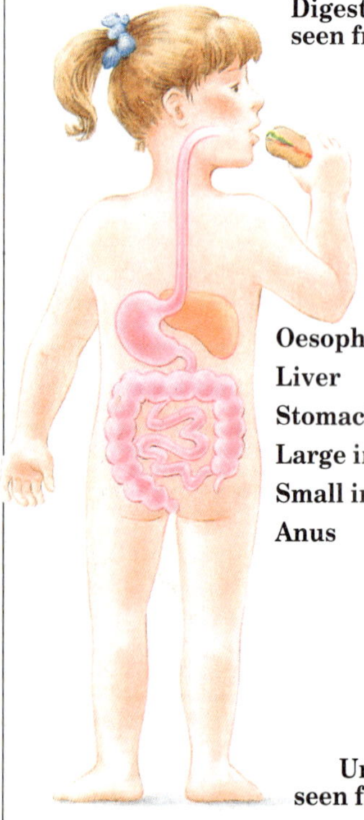

Digestive system seen from the back

Oesophagus
Liver
Stomach
Large intestine
Small intestine
Anus

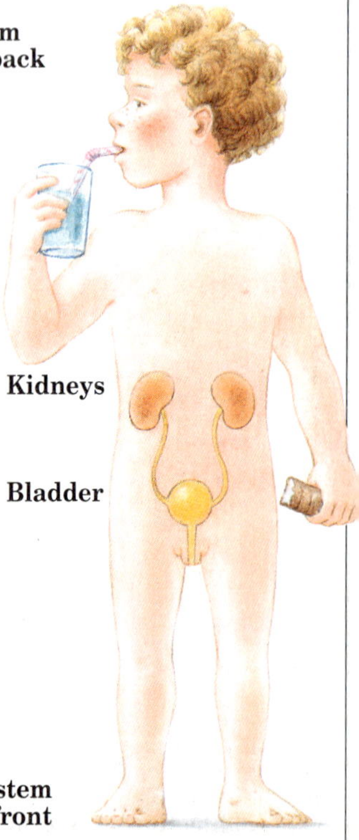

Kidneys

Bladder

Urinary system seen from the front

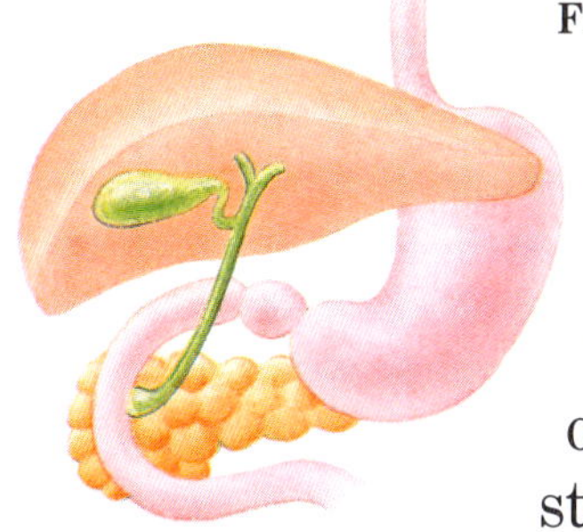

From the liver, a liquid called bile pours into the intestine to help with digestion.

Well chewed and mushy with saliva, food goes down the oesophagus to your stomach. There it is mixed with digestive chemicals into a thick soup. Muscles squeeze it into the small intestine, where useful bits of food called nutrients are separated out and seep into the blood to feed the body's cells. Waste passes into the large intestine and out of the body through the anus. Your blood is cleaned by two filters, your kidneys, which turn any waste products and extra water into urine.

I've got a tummy ache!

Perhaps you've eaten something bad, or you might have an infection, or maybe you're just constipated. Have you drunk enough water?

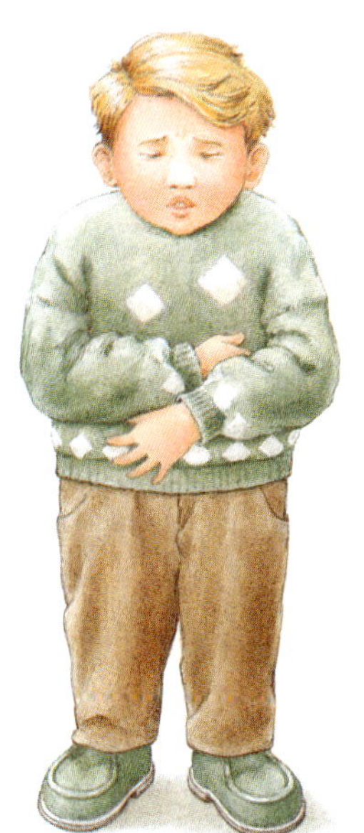

You may hear someone say they've got heartburn. In fact, it's their stomach that's causing the trouble: they've got indigestion.

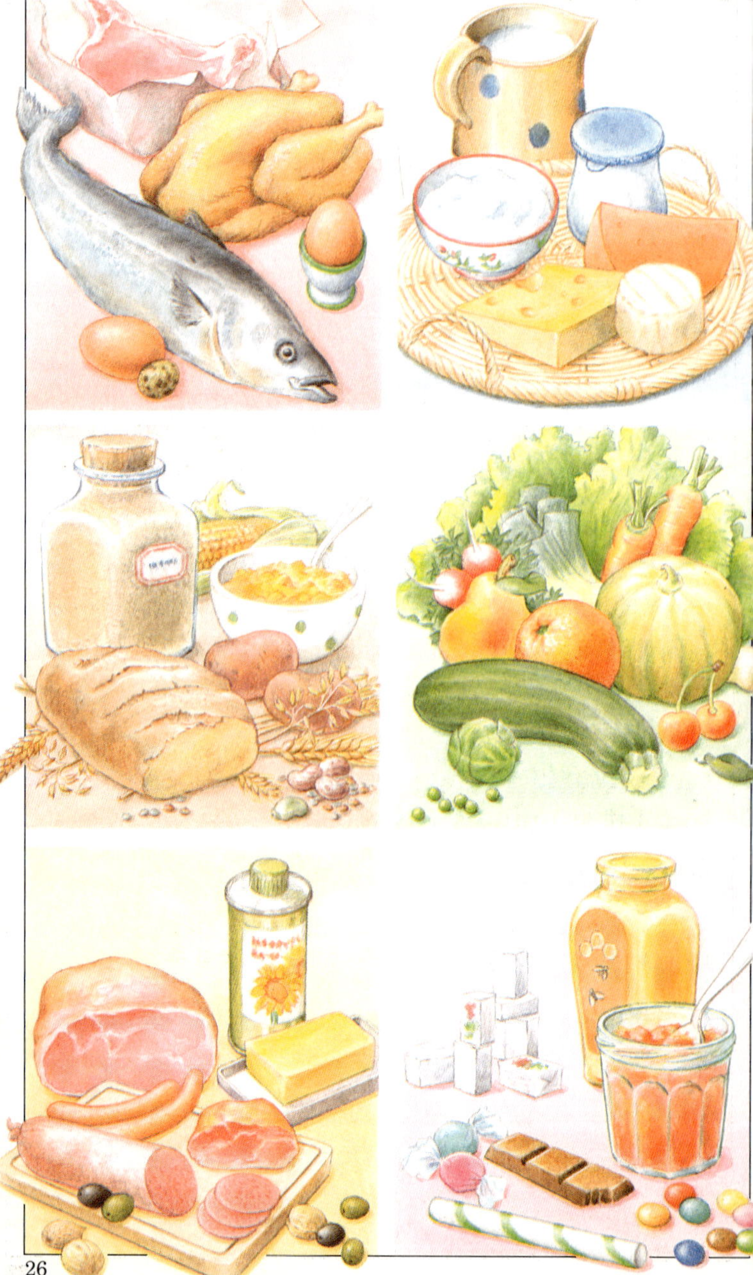

Whilst you are young,
you are growing all the time.
To be strong, your body needs a regular supply of a variety of foods.
It would not work properly if it only had one sort of food. Scientists have shown that we should drink plenty of water, and that our daily meals should include at least one food from each of the following groups: fruit and vegetables give us minerals and vitamins, to help prevent certain diseases, and fibre to keep our digestive system working well. Meat, fish, eggs and dairy products give us protein and are the building blocks of our diet. Bread, rice, potatoes and pasta are carbohydrates and give us energy. Sugar and fat supply us with energy too, but we should not eat too much of them.

Our food comes from many different sources: mineral (water and salt), animal (meat) and vegetable. We are omnivores.

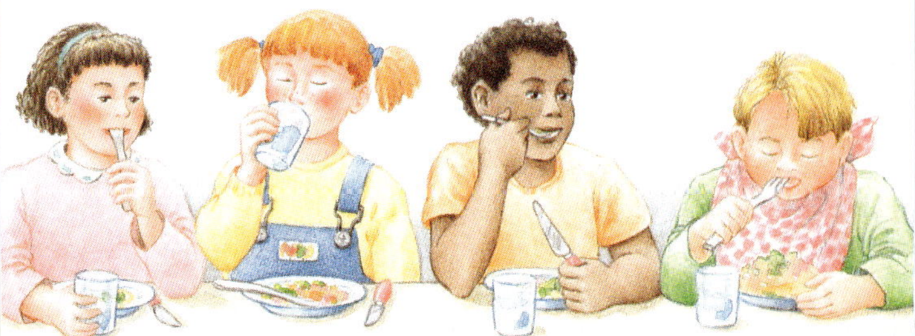

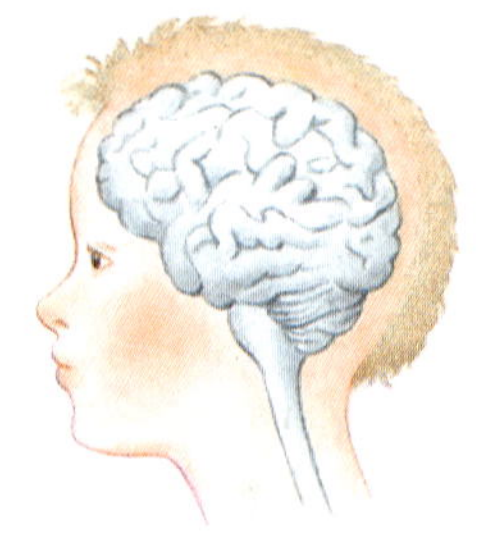

How does everything work so cleverly together in your body?

The brain is the control centre. It is linked to the rest of the body by the spinal cord and a few kilometres of nerves. We call it the nervous system. When you are small, your brain is smooth. Over the years it grows larger and creases, until it weighs about 1.5 kgs and looks like a large walnut. Has anyone ever called you a birdbrain, if you've done something silly? That's because animals have brains which are far less large and developed than yours. Your brain is made up of millions of nerve cells. It works rather like a telephone exchange.

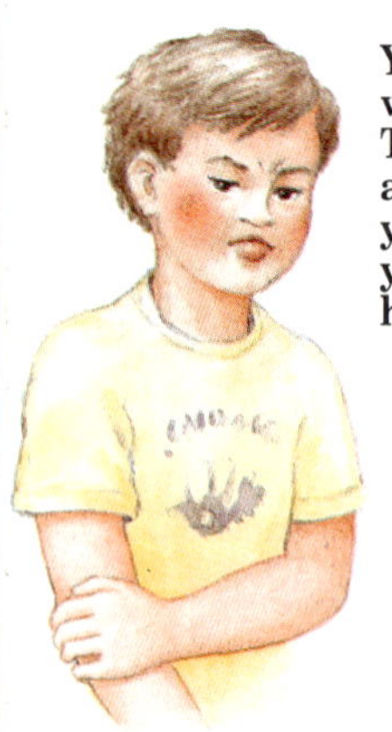

You touch something hot which could burn you. The message arrives at your brain that your hand hurts, and your brain tells your hand to move away!

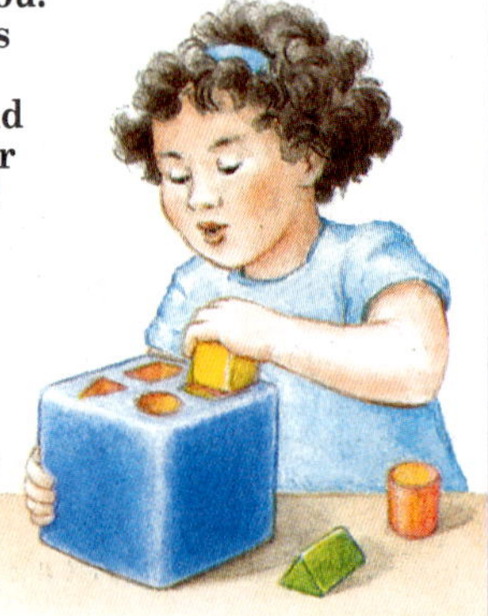

The cube fits into the square hole: the order comes from your brain.

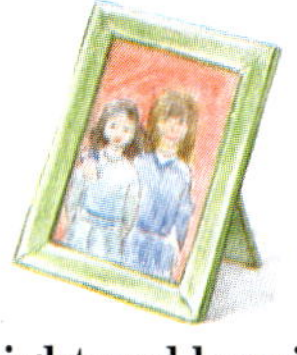
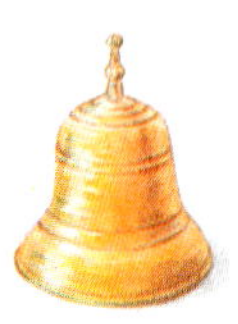

The five senses are smell, taste, touch, sight and hearing. All five are regulated by the brain.

Your brain is sending and receiving thousands of messages, sorting them out and answering them.

Your nerves are the telephone lines which relay these messages. Some are under your control: I want to pick up that pen. Many of them you can't control, like your heart beating, or your lungs working. Memory, thought and feeling are also the brain's work.

Spinal cord

Are you left or right handed?

Your brain is divided into two hemispheres, left and right. Each directs movements on the opposite side of the body. One side is stronger, usually the left, so most people are right-handed. If you are left-handed, the opposite is true.

The spinal cord is like a central cable collecting messages at all levels of the body.

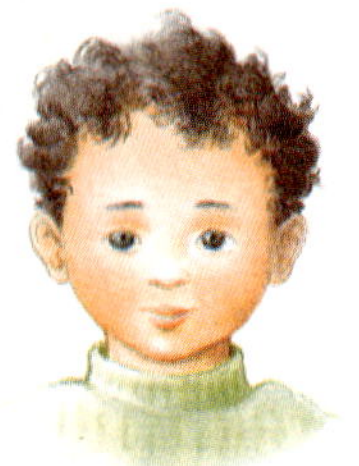
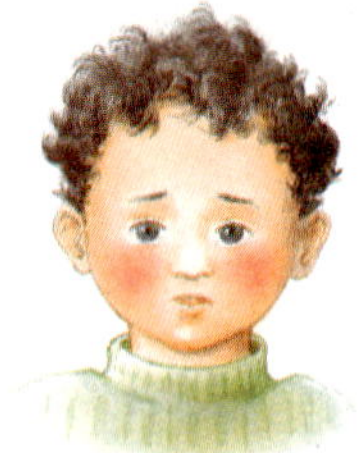
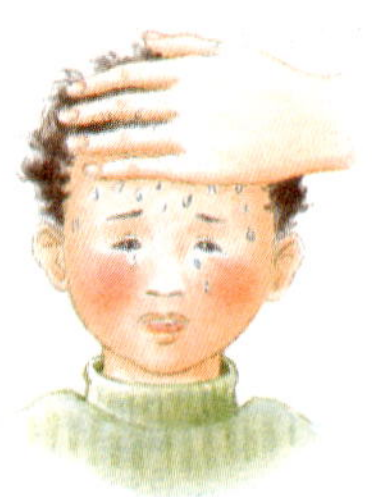

You are shivering, you don't feel well, you have a temperature. These are all signs that you have an infection.

Bacteria and viruses

Germs are the smallest things living on earth, and they affect your body from time to time. Some bacteria are friendly; you need them to help digest food, for instance. Others are enemies. If they break through your defences, they can give you an infection – your body and the germs fight a battle. Your temperature rises because heat can kill off certain germs. If you have a fever, you should drink lots of water to replace lost fluid.

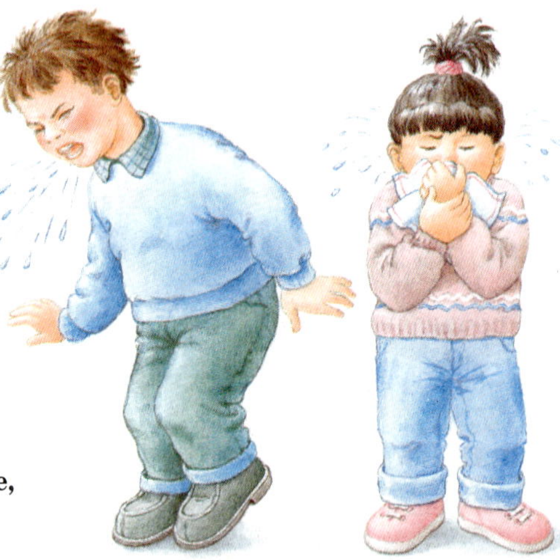

When you cough and sneeze, you are getting rid of germs.

White blood cells go on the attack!

They swallow up germs. Your bone-marrow, which makes blood cells, has to speed up production. Sometimes your body wins on its own. At other times, medicines like antibiotics are given by a doctor to help you. Vaccinations also protect you from lots of illnesses: measles, german measles, mumps and whooping-cough used to be very dangerous, until the invention of vaccines. These are known as childhood illnesses, because you usually get them when you are still a child.

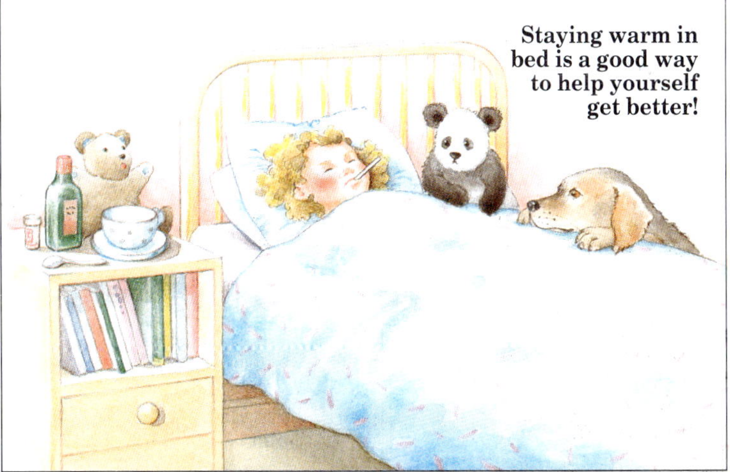

Staying warm in bed is a good way to help yourself get better!

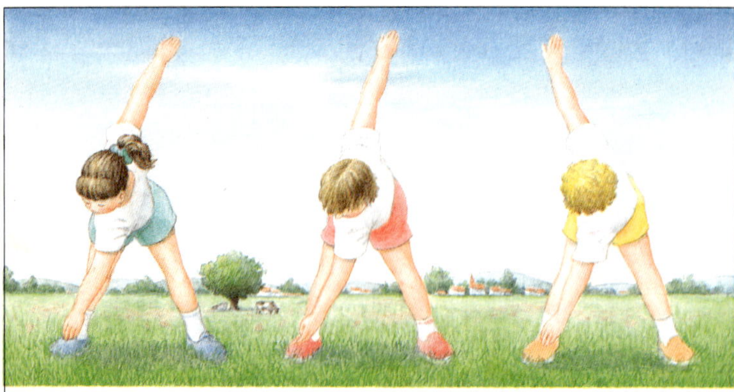

There is nothing like doing a sport that you enjoy.
Physical exercise is vital for a healthy body.

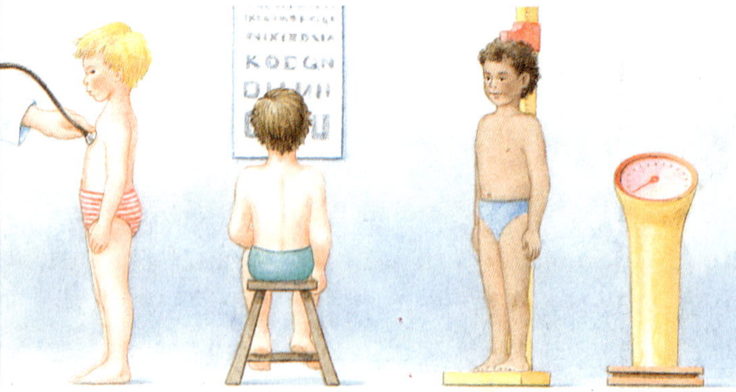

At a child health clinic, your height, weight, and hearing and sight are checked, and vaccinations are given.

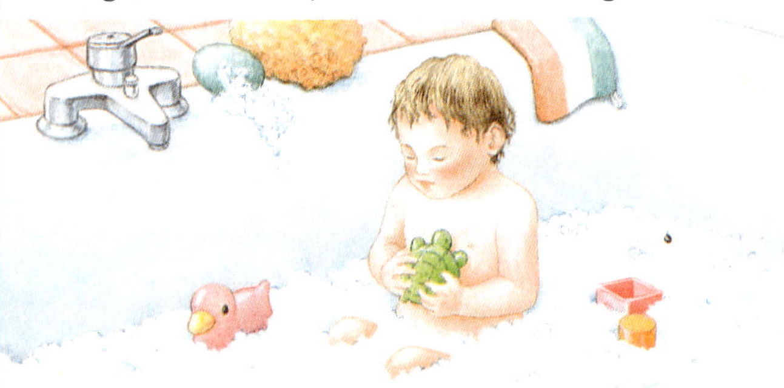

You ought to have a good wash or a bath every day.
And don't forget to brush your teeth regularly!

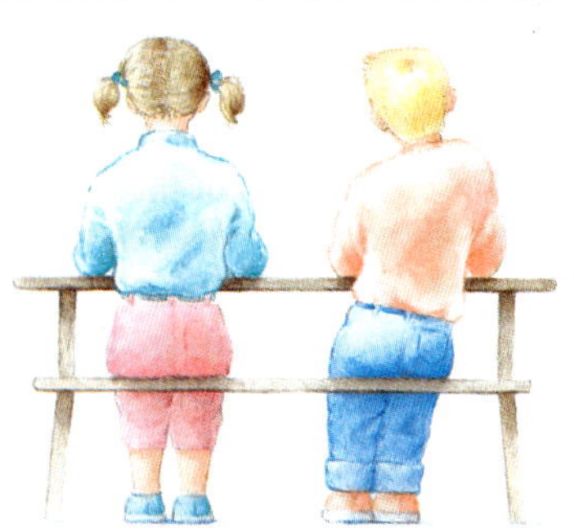

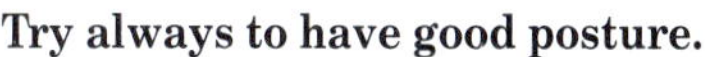

Try always to have good posture.

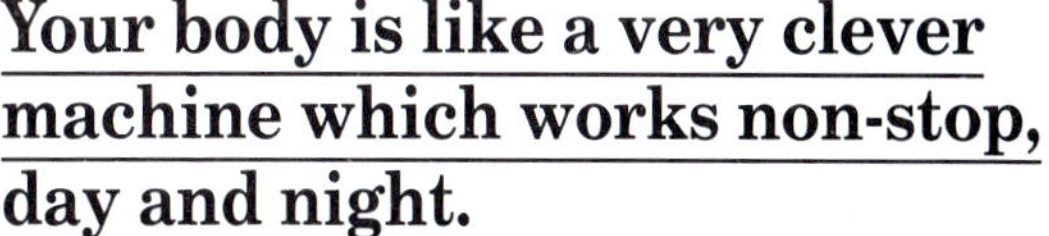

Your body is like a very clever machine which works non-stop, day and night.

It runs beautifully, but occasionally has breakdowns, some more serious than others. You have to mend it. This is normal life, but it helps if you take good care of your machine: eat well, keep clean, take exercise and give yourself enough sleep, so that your body can rest and grow.

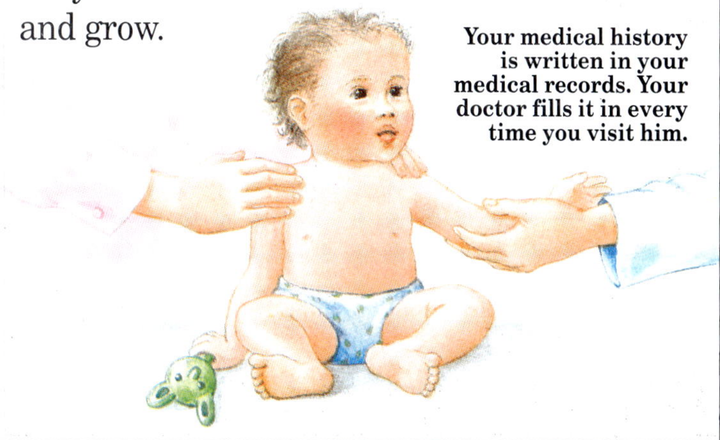

Your medical history is written in your medical records. Your doctor fills it in every time you visit him.

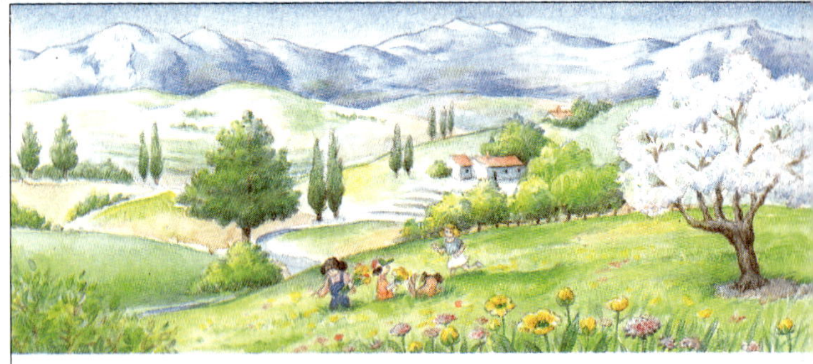

In the spring, the warmer weather and the signs of new life all around us lift our spirits and help us feel energetic.

Rhythms of life

Each person's body has its own built-in rhythm, following the course of day and night, and the seasons, hot and cold. Some people are more active in the evening, and like to get up late in the morning. Others like to get up early. Whether you are a night owl or an early bird, you have to adapt your body's rhythm to fit in with others around you!

In the summer sunshine, our bodies replenish their supplies of Vitamin D. We will need it to help us through the winter.

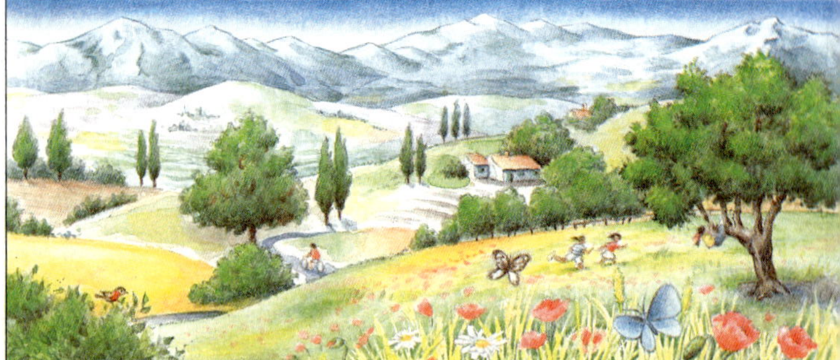

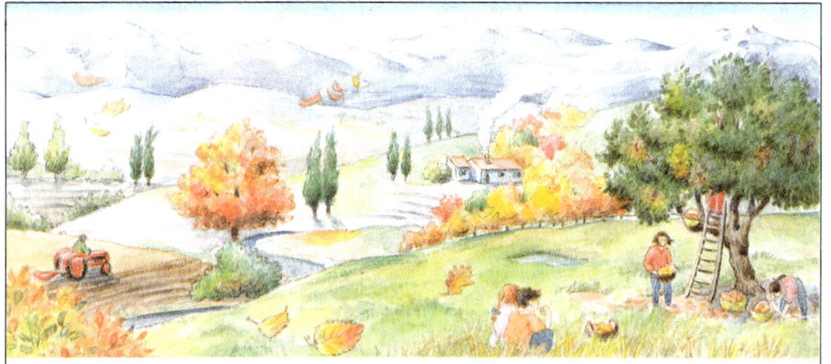

Now it's autumn. Nature slows down. But it's back to school for you, perhaps with a new teacher and a new class.

We spend one third of our lives asleep.

But our brains do not simply 'switch off'. Many things go on in our bodies while we sleep. Dreams help the brain sort out all the ideas, emotions, sights and sounds it has received. Large amounts of growth hormone are produced, to help repair or replace damaged tissue. In the morning, our temperature is always lower. It rises with all the activities we pack into a day.

In winter, some animals hibernate. Some of us would like to sleep all winter too – it's hard to get up on dark mornings!

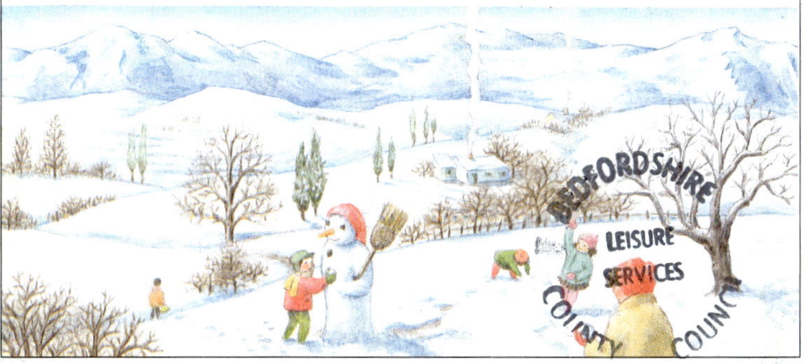

Index

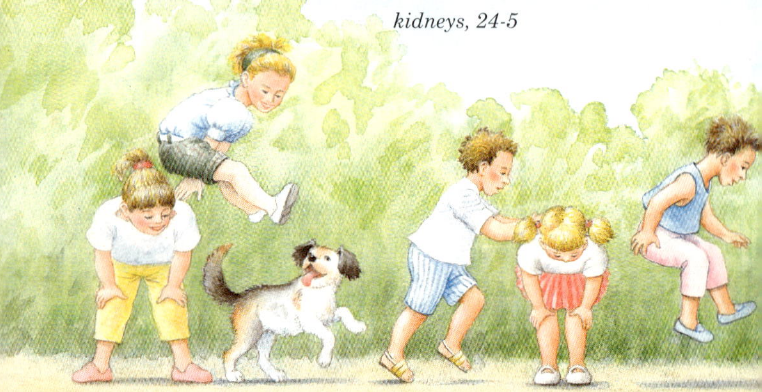

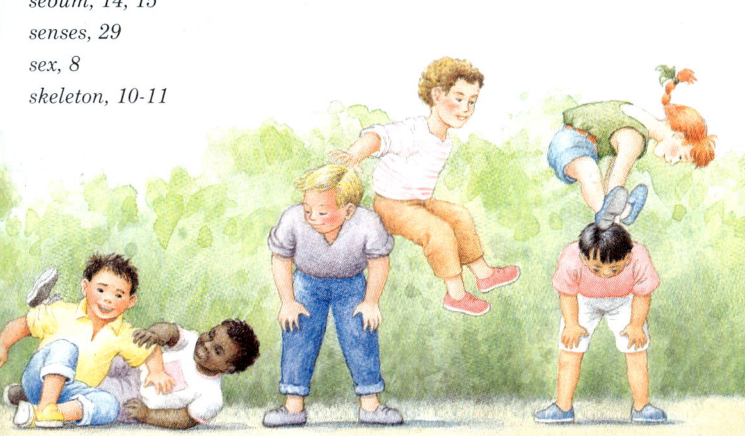

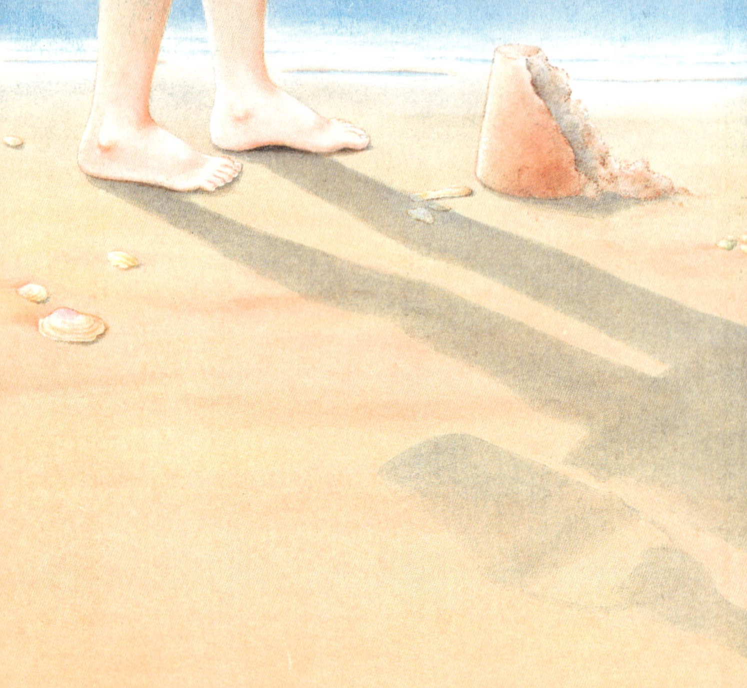

Pocket Worlds – building up into a child's first encyclopaedia:

The Human World
Living in Ancient Egypt
Living in Ancient Greece
Living in Ancient Rome
Living with the Eskimos
Living in the Sahara
Living in India
Living on a Tropical Island
Living in Australia
Living in the Heart of Africa
On the Trail of the American Indians
Cowboys and Pioneers
The Building of the Great Cathedrals
Long Ago in a Castle
The Other Side of the Screen
Firemen to the Rescue
The Making of Music
The Story of Writing
People Who Work While We Sleep
Bridges, Tunnels and Towers
Transport Yesterday and Today
The Long and Rich History of Trade
Money Through the Ages
Measuring the World
Sleep and Dreams
Your Body
The Five Senses
The Story of Birth and Babies